Natural Hair Recipes For Moisture and Growth

Step By Step Instructions On How

To Create and Apply Conditioners,

Creams, Oils, and Treatments For

Dry, Curly, Kinky Afrocentric Hair

Argena Hall

www.NaturalHairMaster.com

Natural Hair Checklist & Journal [FREE]

Our printable checklist provides you with a list of everything you'll need to begin your natural hair journey.

Take it with you on the go, it can be downloaded on any device.

As an added **BONUS** you'll receive our **Natural Hair Journey Journal**. A digital journal where you can track your experiences of growth, recipes, and more.

www.naturalhairmaster.com/naturalhairchecklistandjournal

Table of Contents

GETTING TO KNOW YOUR HAIR

Your hair isn't growing. It's dry and breaking off like dead leaves in the winter time. It's rough to the touch and seems like just about every time you style it, you come away with a mound of broken strands about the size of a small lemon, sometimes more but hopefully less! As you start and continue on the journey to regain the health of your kinky, curly hair, there are many things to consider. From hair growth and loss, to keeping your strands as long as possible; one of the most prevalent issues affecting our kinky, coiled hair is keeping it moist and damage free. The following recipes will help ease the process to gaining a healthier head of hair.

However, before we delve into the recipes, let's take some time to answer a few questions that will give you some insight toward the causes of hair growth, loss, and how moisture retention will help your progress along this journey.

HOW DOES HAIR GROW

Some of the things that one needs to know, when it comes to the actual growing of hair, is it's structure and the pattern in which it grows. Hair develops via two different structures - the follicle can be found in the skin, buried in the scalp, and second, the hair we see growing out of our heads.

The tubular portion of the strand is actually the strand which nestles down deep beneath the skin's surface. It contains several layers, and each layer serves a different purpose. The papilla is the first layer, which contains capillaries that carry blood, cultivating and nurturing the cells. The bulb is a layer that lives and breathes, and it surrounds the papilla and is right near the surface of the scalp waiting to assist your hair in it's growing process. Extending out and surrounding the follicle are an inner and outer strand, the cuticle of the hair. The inner casing follows the hair helping to develop curl patterns and ends right on the edge of a scent gland, or a sebaceous gland, which is more widely known for secreting oil. There is an erector pili muscle that forms around the bottom of the follicle and when it squeezes on tight, it forces the sebum out onto the hair and scalp. The natural oil secreted by the sebaceous gland is necessary to the conditioning of our skin and nails.

All of that luxurious hair atop of your head is actually created from keratin which is a dead protein, a three layered, hardened, dead protein to be exact. The medulla, the cortex, and the cuticle form that wonderful hair band called Keratin. The leader of this group is the cortex which hogs the fame as most of the hair shaft is developed from this layer. Cuticle is doing backup, making those tightly formed, overlapping scales, similar to roof shingles. While the medulla is rounding out the trio helping to bring color to this group and to your hair.

Understanding the composition of each strand will give you a better understanding when it comes to your particular hair. Now consider how it grows. The average person can see about seven to nine inches of hair growth within a year. However, periods of growth and shedding vary from person to person. Your hair cycle flows in three separate stages, which are the anagen, catagen, and telogen. Unfortunately, every strand doesn't have to be in the same stage at the same time. This may be why you notice one side of your head grows longer and faster than the other. The anagen stage is when your scalp just can't seem to stop itching! It's growing baby. Those shingle-like scales of the hair are splitting and piling onto each other rapidly. A new hair makes room for itself and pushes the hair that is no longer in the growth phase up through the deep layers of your skin and out of the scalp, which results in the length of your hair. Hair will grow abundantly or very little during this stage, but most average about half a centimeter every month. And again, this varies between individual scalps. Your hair can actually be in this replenishing state for two to six years. Some years are better than others for our scalps, and there are several outlying factors that contribute to this, which are gone over in a later section. Naturally, it makes more sense that the shorter your anagen phase the shorter your hair and vice versa.

The catagen period can affect up to some five percent of hair at any given time. This part of the hair cycle is when each strand has to be told to stop growing before the shedding can begin.

Lastly, about 8-11 % of your hair will be shedding in the telogen stage of your hair cycle. It lasts for about 110 days for hairs on the scalp. Growth and all of the itchiness associated with such should be subdued as you scalp and hair follicles are to be resting during this period. If you ever lose a strand at the root during this time, you'll see that solid, hard, white bulb clinging to the bottom. One can expect to lose about 22 to 115 of these hairs daily during this phase. Good thing we have so many.

WHAT CAUSES HAIR GROWTH & LOSS

Soft, moisturized hair isn't enjoyable if you're constantly losing it. Whether it falls out or breaks off, pay attention to some signs of hair loss prior to jumping into an entirely new hair care regimen. Figuring out if there's a problem and/ or what the problem is, is way better than trying a bunch of solutions that band aid a more serious issue.

Stress can be one of the culprits to hair loss. One of the most common types of stress to cause hair to shed is telogen effluvium. Effluvium means outflow, and telogen is the hair's natural shedding phase so you can only imagine the increased amount of strands leaving your scalp when under stressful situations. Try some stress relieving exercises that may temporarily ease the pressure because stress not only affects your hair, but your overall physical and mental health.

Our internal health can also wreak havoc on our follicles. The duties performed by our hormones are regulated by the thyroid, so as the largest endocrine gland, when it's not in tip top shape prepare for life altering effects. When the thyroid starts acting up, many of us suffer from severe hair loss. Whether it's producing too many hormones or not enough, when this particular gland is out of whack, many will experience hair loss, thinning, and even dry hair.

Sometimes illness intruders affect our bodies. Intruders like cancer and polycystic ovary syndrome. From their treatments to the actual disorders themselves, problems with hair loss from the scalp arise in many women. They can also cause fertility problems, irregular periods and severe thinning of hair on the scalp.

Be sure that if you notice any significant changes in the density or shedding of your. hair that you seek medical attention, whether it be from a dermatologist or your primary care physician. But, that's enough stress about losing our hair, let's check out some ways to help it grow and retain the length of your choosing.

Make sure to keep your ends trimmed, to keep them healthy. While that may seem a bit contradictory when it comes to keeping your hair long, if you want healthy long hair you need to get regular trims. Those split ends promote breakage, hair loss, and weaken the healthy hair growing out near your scalp. So keep it neat and tidy and trim those ends.

Utilize the natural oils of your scalp by giving yourself a nice scalp massage at night. Or have someone massage it for you, if you don't mind another person's set of hands in your hair. Whether it be with a brush or your fingertips, spreading around your body's natural oils will do wonders to promote growth and lock in moisture. You can keep your scalp so much healthier by doing this one simple step every night. Speaking of your scalp, think of it in terms of nature. Trees can't grow if the soil and roots aren't taken care of, so treat your hair similarly. Healthy hair starts with a healthy scalp, which will make it easier for your hair to stay moisturized. You can do a quick and easy test to see how healthy your hair and scalp is. Take a section of your hair and lift it at the root. Healthier hair holds the same density from the root to the tip. If your ends are thinner, you may want to utilize some of the following treatments to stimulate a healthier hair care regimen. Or you may be at a point where it's best for you to just chop it off and start over. It's only hair it'll grow back.

The best way to start a new hair healthcare regimen is from the inside by eating the right foods, and adding a daily vitamin to that as well. Nothing promotes a luxurious mane like eating right. It makes you feel and look good from the inside out. Keep in mind to look for multivitamins that are formulated for hair skin and nails, which often contain biotin, vitamin C and those essential B vitamins.

While we love for our hair to look phenomenal, be careful not to overdo it with the heat styling tools. Don't over style your hair as excessive heat can lead to damage and unnecessary breakage. Along with excessive heat, you're going to want to skip the excessive shampooing as well. Our afrocentric hair can go weeks without a wash but it is recommended to wash once a week or every two weeks. As the days without shampooing pass, your natural oils build up and penetrate your hair allowing for it to hydrate and repair some of the damage on its own. However, if you go too long without a good scrub the buildup will cause itching, flaking, and dandruff. That kind of itching ain't the hair growth phase. And when it comes time to wash that buildup away, use cool water to rinse so it can help seal the cuticles and protect your hair while styling it. Once you're styled and ready for bed, take care to sleep on a silk pillowcase. Silk tends to be less damaging on the hair avoiding tangles and breakage. The less breakage the longer and healthier the hair.

Last, but not least, pay attention to how your skin and scalp react after using certain products. There are many signs to look out for that a product isn't working for you. Even if your hair shiny, if the product leaves your skin feeling dry, waxed, stripped, or even worse irritated (bumps, itching, or hives), seek medical attention if necessary and reconsider what you're putting onto your hair.

So now that we've touched on the basics of structure, growth, and loss; let's move on to keeping the strands moisturized. Moisturizing the hair isn't exactly what keeps the hair growing, it keeps the strands strong during styling so you can avoid damage and breakage. But the absolute key to locking in moisture, especially if your hair is naturally dry, is to make it routine. Here are a few things to always keep in the house when you want to whip up a few of these recipes. Just by keeping a few of these staples on hand, you can alter and change these recipes as you discover what works for your hair and what does not.

KEEP THESE IN THE HOUSE

As previously mentioned, many of the following recipes will use one or more of the following items and even if you don't follow these recipes to the letter, you can mix and match the ingredients below into a product that your hair will love. Take care to learn if you are allergic to any of the products and steer clear, but otherwise, mix, match, and find what works best for your coiled strands.

Many conditioner and moisturizer recipes start off with some kind of conditioner base. The creamier the better. **Thick**

conditioners, avocado, or even mayonnaise can be used as they promote shine and moisture retention.

Some liquids to keep on hand, which keep the hair shaft soft, are **aloe vera juice, glycerin, and/or water. Aloe Vera Juice** moisturizes and helps your curly strands blossom, but it also provides remarkable sheen by securing oil into the hair channel. **Glycerin** conditions by binding water together and other ingredients to amplify your mane's moisture level. And **water** of course, can't be left off of this list as it's readily available to many of us and is the holy grail of moisturizing liquid since our body requires it for basic survival.

There are tons of oils on the market, but here are just a few that you can use to lock the above liquids into the hair. **Argan Oil** is often considered "liquid diamonds" which leaves your hair softer, smoother, and glistening. **Avocado Oil** is perfect for saving parched, damaged hair, or relieving an irritated scalp. **Coconut Oil** is great for soaking in moisture as it's not easily broken down or evaporated. It also keeps your hair strong and soft and aiding in the prevention of hair shedding and thinning. **Extra Virgin Olive Oil** also locks in moisture and soothes dry and itchy scalp, resulting in shiny, beautiful hair. **Jojoba Oil** is one of the oils closer to your body's naturally produced oil, sebum, which will be well absorbed by your coils.

Now to seal the oil and moisture into the hair shaft a good sealant to keep around is some **Shea Butter**. Shea butter protects the hair against the harsh elements of the seasons, softens the hair, and soothes an irritated scalp. Any emollient can be used to seal in the liquid and oils. So you can choose from your favorite leave-in conditioner, hair dressing lotion, and even butters like shea, cocoa, or even mango.

Keeping a few of these products in the house will always help when you're in a bind and can't get out to the store to get some much needed ingredients for your wash day routine. So let's put these ingredients to work. Moving through the wash day is the simplest way to convey some really fun recipes that will help moisturize and grow your hair. Let's start with the Pre Poo.

PRE POO RECIPES FOR YOU

Prior to shampooing or conditioning your hair, you can develop a concoction of sorts to help moisturize your locks as you move through your wash day routine. Therefore the name comes from just that, pre-shampoo to prepoo. It helps protect the strands against the hazardous stripping of shampooing, drying, and styling. Layering these steps will promote healthy strong hair and scalp.

PRE POO RECIPES

Here are nine pre poo recipes that you can use on any given wash day. The ingredients are definitely interchangeable and can be altered to your hair's liking.

1. Avocado PrePoo — A favorite among many naturalistas, this basic recipe is easy to make and easy to work through your hair.

Ingredients:

1 RIPE Hass Avocado (Must be ripe and soft so when you blend it you aren't left with tiny

chunks that will cling to your strands and leave you utterly frustrated when you try to remove them)

2.5 Tablespoons of Coconut Oil (Feel free to add other oils in addition to this. Only result will be a thinner mask)

Directions

Cut the avocado in half, peel it, and cut avocado into small pieces.

Place the ingredients in a blender and mix thoroughly. You want it to be the consistency of something similar to condensed milk or a thick conditioner. The blender is best as it eliminates those chunks that may be left behind if you choose to mix with a fork or other utensil.

Heating the mixture prior to application will help in spreading through the scalp.

Section your hair in however many manageable sections you prefer. You can separate your hair with your fingers if you don't particularly like combs.

Go through each section, from root tip, coating your hair with the mixture until your entire head is covered. Saving any leftovers from this mixture is not recommended but can be done by placing in air-tight container and into the fridge but must be used within a few days.

Cover your hair with a plastic cap, for at least 40 minutes.

Rinse with warm water and proceed with wash day regimen.

2. Olive Oil Cover – It's very simple and easy to complete, and uses one of those staples mentioned above. It can work when you're in a pinch for time and will leave your hairs luxuriously elastic and increase the moisture and strength of your hair while washing.

Ingredients:

2/3 cup Extra Virgin Olive Oil (Feel free to cut this with another oil to save yourself from running out quickly)

3 Tablespoons Honey (Raw Honey is best but any store bought honey will do)

Directions:

Blend the two ingredients together resulting in a luxurious liquid.

Section your hair into sections suitable for you to handle. You can separate your hair with your fingers instead of a comb.

Go through each section, from root tip, coating your hair with the mixture until your entire head is covered.

Cover your hair with a plastic shower cap, or any cover to stop the oil from running down the side of face, for no longer than 42 minutes. You can wrap it with a towel to heat it up or sit under a hooded dryer to open up the cuticle allowing the oil to really soak into the shaft.

Rinse with cool water and proceed with wash day regimen.

3. Coconut Milk Smoothie PrePoo – If you happen to have some left over from all those delicious smoothies you make, this mask can deliver a delightful head of soft, shiny, moisturized hair.

Ingredients:

½ cup Coconut Milk (Do not confuse this for coconut oil or any sweetened coconut milk based product)

1 ripe avocado

2 tablespoons Olive Oil

2 tablespoons of honey

Directions:

Peel and cut the avocado into pieces or halves.

Using a blender will eliminate the chunks from the avocado or use the back of a spoon to mash out the chunky pieces.

Section your hair with a comb or your fingers to ease the mixture through your coils.

Go through each section, from root tip, coating your hair with the mixture until your entire head is covered.

You can wrap it with a towel to heat it up or sit under a hooded dryer after you cover with a cap; no longer than 34minutes.

Rinse with cool water and proceed with wash day regimen.

4. Shea butter – For less moisturizing upkeep during the week, this pre poo can be used on wash day as well.

Ingredients:

2/3 cup Shea Butter

1 tablespoon Extra Virgin Olive Oil

1 tablespoon Coconut Oil

1 tablespoon Castor Oil

2 tablespoons Honey

Directions:

You're going to warm these ingredients together prior to mixing.

Since this mixture isn't as thick as the others you're going to want to apply this as quickly as possible to avoid oil running down your temples and forehead. Saturate the hair and cover for 45 minutes.

Rinse with cool water and proceed with wash day regimen.

5. Banana Mask – A banana mask requires a blender, much like the avocado, to relieve you of fruit chunks clinging to your hair and the painstaking process of removing them later.

Ingredients

1 Ripe banana (That bruised and brown banana left in the bunch that no one in the house wants to eat is one way to get rid of it without wasting food or money.)

3 tablespoons Extra Virgin Olive Oil (Cut or replace with any oil of your choice)

2 tablespoons Honey

Directions:

Peel the banana and discard the peel (or use it to polish leather, it's supposed to be good for that)

Blend well. Make sure there aren't any chunks left in the mixture.

Slather onto hair and scalp, concentrating on the ends. Cover for at least 30 minutes and rinse with lukewarm water.

6. Commercial Conditioner – Sometimes simplicity is key. Using a cheap conditioner you already have available in the house is easy to use without much mixing involved.

Ingredients:

1 cup conditioner

2 ½ tablespoons of an essential oil (Feel free to mix it up and add the oils your hair loves here)

Directions:

Mix well, saturate the hair, and cover for an hour. Rinse the conditioner out and move on to your next step.

7. Mango PrePoo – Is an emollient as well as a great base for any of these pre poo recipes, in case you dislike avocado, or just don't have any in the house. It has a very thick consistency and works wonders when blended with some of your other staple ingredients.

Ingredients:

½ cup Mango Butter

½ cup Shea Butter

3 tablespoons Coconut Oil

1.5 Tablespoon Honey

Directions:

If you don't want to churn butter for minutes on end, make it easier to mix by warming the butter before you use them. Heat the butters, but not too hot as this is going to be applied to your scalp and hair. 30 – 45 seconds in the microwave should be enough to get the butters more malleable. Or you can let the butters sit in a hot water bath until they soften enough for you to use.

Section your hair and coat each strand tip to root, or root to tip, whichever you prefer.

Cover your hair and let those luxurious scents absorb into your hair.

Rinse with cool water and proceed with wash day regimen.

8. Egg Wash PrePoo – This protein rich mask is known to work wonders on your curls, especially if you just took out a protective style and need an extra boost of protein to your coils.

Ingredients:

1 Egg

½ cup plain Greek yogurt

1 tablespoon Mayonnaise (this doesn't have to be added but is great for additional protein)

2 tablespoons of Oil (any essential oil of your choice will suffice)

Directions:

Blending this mixture in a blender may leave you with a frothy, foamy type mixture, so to avoid that an egg beater is suggested to keep a creamy consistency.

Section your hair with a rat tail, or wide tooth comb.

Go through each section, from root tip, coating your hair with the mixture until your entire head is covered.

Cover your hair with a plastic shower cap for 20-45 minutes.

Rinse with cool or cold water to avoid scrambled eggs in your hair.

9. Castor Oil PrePoo - Castor oil is thick enough to encase and infiltrate the hair shaft helping to lessen dryness, stray hairs, and safeguard against the harsh stripping properties of cleansers. You may balk at the price of castor oil and extra virgin olive oil so it's best to use these oils with other to prolong their usage. You can also use Jamaican Black Castor Oil as a substitute for regular castor oil. There is a description explaining the difference between the two following the recipe.

Ingredients:

¼ cup Castor Oil

2 tablespoons Honey

1 tablespoon Almond Oil

2 tablespoons Mayonnaise

Directions:

Mix the ingredients well and apply to hair and scalp. Cover your hair with a plastic cap for a minimum of 30 minutes and rinse it out.

THE DIFFERENCE BETWEEN CASTOR OIL & JAMAICAN BLACK CASTOR OIL

Regular castor oil can be bought just about anywhere and is more popular than its counterpart, Jamaican Black Castor Oil (JBCO). Castor oil has a pale yellow hue and is often priced slightly lower than JBCO. Castor oil that isn't altered by heat or any other substances is why they refer to it as *cold pressed*. The lighter the hue and clearer the oil means the oil is closer to its purest form. This pure form is just as good as the standard, except that the iodine has been removed, which is what gives it the yellowish hue.

JBCO is a very dark color as the nut, from which castor oil is derived from, is roasted and then the ashes are added back into the pressed oil. This oil has been said to have a very potent scent, so less is definitely more when applying this oil to your hair. JBCO generally costs more than regular castor oil and it can be hard to find as beauty supply stores and websites tend to be its only suppliers. You will probably find regular castor oil in your neighborhood drug stores but it's helpful to do a price comparison before choosing which one you would like to use. They are interchangeable in any of these recipes that require the use of castor oil.

There isn't enough scientific evidence to prove that JBCO is the better version, even though many coiled divas swear it's the holy grail of their hair care regimen, often toted as a hair growth stimulant especially for those trouble areas around the nape and temples. The ash that's been added to the JBCO is said to act like a super fertilizer for the scalp, which leads many to believe that the darker or blacker the oil, the better. All in all, you can use either version of the oil as they have both had similar effects and benefits in the growth of hair and

conditioning.

ENTER DEEP CONDITIONING

Speaking of conditioning, let's move along passed the pre poo, after your shampoo, and into deep conditioning. There are certainly many questions that come to mind when instituting your deep condition treatment. Does it have to be left in for so long? Does it have to be a set time limit for different recipes? Should it be with laced with protein or advocate moisture? Do the cheap ones work just as good as the expensive ones? Can and should you use food to deep condition? Let's answer that last one with a resounding yes because some of the recipes provided will have some edible components.

Now for a successful deep condition, that will help your hair lock in that softness and moisture, here are some tips of the essential do's and don'ts you may want to think about.

Heat up your deep conditioner if you want it working overtime to make your hair feel super plush, strong, and luxurious. 95 degrees Fahrenheit heightens the amount and outcome of absorption for that conditioner. A hot water bath tends to work better than the microwave when heating your deep conditioner prior to its application.

Switching up your conditioners, from protein based to moisture based, will keep your coily strands soft, strong, and healthy which will help along the journey to solidifying its moisture and length. Some ingredients to pay attention to in your conditioners are cetyl, stearyl, and cetearyl for additional softness. If they contain butters and oils along with products that absorb water from the environment to add into your hairs, like vegetable glycerin and aloe vera, your hair will be full of nutrients and everything else it needs to stay soft with a healthy bounce. Look for proteins like keratin, amino acids, and henna if you want a treatment fortified for strength. After applying the deep conditioner, don't rush to get out of the bathroom. That steam, which has built up, is perfect for penetrating the hair. But if you want to save water, and some money on your utility bill, invest in a steamer or hooded dryer to sit under to let cuticle lift and open up, allowing for absorption of the treatment. When applying the treatment, start with your ends. This will allow the treatment time to infiltrate them longer while you work up toward your scalp.

Don't obsess over the price. Compare ingredients between expensive brands and cheaper drugstore brands, and if the cheaper brand has a similar composition then go for what's best for your wallet. Splurge if you like but don't be fooled by products promising magic hair growth or quick fix solutions to your dry, brittle hair. Pay attention to the components as the first four to six ingredients are the most potent and do the actual work within the product. You can even use some of these recipes to bridge the gap between buys. Do not keep these natural, food containing mixtures stored for long though. They don't have any preservatives like store bought products to prolong their lifespan. Use your mixtures within a few days and refrigerate up to five days max.

Now while you're waiting for your deep conditioner to activate and seep into your kinky coils, you don't want to overdo it. Hours on end or overnight deep conditioning treatments are unnecessary, unless the instructional use of a particular product dictate otherwise. Let your conditioner do the work without it consuming your entire day. Half an hour should be enough. Again, let your deep conditioner do the job you bought it for. Don't use it as a leave-in or as a deep conditioning treatment. Deep conditioners have particular elements designed to cling to your strands for permeation, which can leave your tresses feeling heavy and limp if you use it any other way.

When you deep condition your hair regularly, it's more manageable, it's softer, it doesn't break off as easy which correlates to less frizz and it's better able to retain its length. But, you determine what regularly is. That can be from every three to four days to every two weeks, but at least once a week would be optimal. See how your hair reacts to the frequency. For instance, if your hair feels super saturated (meaning it's never quite dry), limp, or weak, you're conditioning too often and try lessening it to every 2 weeks. However, if it begins to feel too dry and lackluster you may want to increase the treatment to twice a week until your hair gets the resilience you're looking for.

Now let's get into some of these recipes your locks are bound to love. Remember to take care to understand what your hair likes, and if you're allergic to any of the ingredients omit them or substitute them for something you can tolerate.

DEEP CONDITIONER RECIPES

1. **Avocado & Banana Deep Conditioner** – Your hair is in for a real treat once you combine these ingredients into a luxurious deep conditioning masque.

Ingredients:

1 ripe hass avocado

½ ripe banana (or you can use one of those small containers of baby food fruit. Go organic if you use this over an actual banana)

½ cup Coconut Milk

¼ cup mayonnaise

3 tablespoons Honey

Directions:

Remove the avocado and banana from the peel. Cut them into pieces, and add a spoonful of water for easier blending.

You are definitely going to want your blender out for this or churn, churn, churn away until all the chunks are gone. Remember if you don't get the chunks out now, you'll be pulling them out, along with your hair, later.

Apply the deep conditioner treatment to your ends first and move toward the scalp. After the mixture has covered your strands, cover the entire head for no less than a half hour. Rinse with cool to cold water and wash, wash, wash it out thoroughly. Then proceed with styling.

2. **Honey & Avocado for Damaged Hair** – As previously mentioned, your hair has to fend off a lot to stay at its healthiest and it needs a little bit of help from you. Dry, frizzy, frayed ends, dead

ends, split ends, heat damage; all take away from the look and actual health of your hair. Here's a deep condition to help ease your hair's pain.

Ingredients:

1 ripe Avocado

1 tablespoon Honey

1 tablespoon Coconut oil

¼ cup warm Water

Directions:

Don't forget to peel and cut the avocado into small, mixable portions. Blend these ingredients in your blender for a smooth chunk-less concoction.

Lightly coat your strands with the mixture and leave on for about 8 to 12 minutes then rinse off completely with cold water.

Dry your hair well and style as usual.

3. Egg & Coconut Oil – Coconut oil is one of those staples many natural hair curly girls swear by. That is probably because it can be used for so many different functions, from the hair, skin, and nails to cooking. The egg is great as it provides some protein to the treatment for strengthening your strands.

Ingredients:

½ cup Coconut Oil (You can cut this with another oil and its best to sit your coconut oil in a hot water bath until it becomes a liquid)

1 egg

Directions:

Mix the ingredients together but DO NOT do so while the oil is hot as it will cook the egg.

Apply the deep conditioner treatment to your ends first and move toward the scalp. After the mixture has covered your strands, cover the entire head for no less than a half hour.

Rinse thoroughly with COLD water, again so you don't cook the egg, and proceed with styling.

You can use less oil if you just want to treat the ends of your hair rather than the entire head.

4. Avocado & Egg Hair Mask

Ingredients:

1 ripe Avocado

1 egg

Directions:

Peel and cut your avocado in half, throw it into a blender, and crack your egg into the blender as well.

Pulse it until you get a smooth and lump-free avocado egg hair mask.

Apply to your ends working your way slowly up to the roots and scalp.

Leave the hair mask to absorb for at least 9 to 15 minutes.

Rinse with cold water several times to remove the mask and the smell, and towel dry your hair for best results.

Remember that it is always best to blend your fruits and foods in a blender for any and all hair treatments to avoid the chunky bits from sticking to your strands. Hair has enough external elements to fight against, from the environment to heat styling tools, without you purposely afflicting it with the fine tooth comb and wrath of removing fruit bit chunks.

5. Avocado & Olive Oil –This deep conditioning treatment will make your smooth and silky since both avocadoes and olive oil contain fatty acids which lock in moisture, strengthen the strands, and encourage hair growth.

Ingredients:

½ Avocado

¼ cup warm water

1 tablespoon Extra Virgin Olive Oil

2 tablespoons Honey

Directions:

Peel and cut the avocado.

Get out your blender for this one too and mix these four ingredients together until they form a chunk free puree.

Apply to your hair. Wrap your ends in a bun, or several, and cover. Rinse with warm to cold water and proceed with styling.

6. Extra Virgin Olive Oil & Honey – Great as a deep conditioner, and a PrePoo too. The not using your deep conditioner as anything else, mentioned above, is meant for store bought treatments.

Ingredients:

¼ cup Honey

¼ cup Extra Virgin Olive Oil

2 tablespoons Castor Oil

Directions:

Apply the deep conditioner treatment to your ends first and move toward the scalp. After the mixture has covered your strands, cover the entire head for no less than a half hour.

Rinse with warm water and proceed with styling.

Try to use pure, cold pressed oils, and organic products when making your at-home conditioners and pre poo treatments.

Hopefully these deep conditioning treatments are everything and more for your tresses, especially if you live in a climate with colder winters. It is super important, critical even, that you formulate a hair care routine that you can stick to so your hair can keep its moisture and hold onto its length. If you find things aren't working in your favor, or to your liking, it's okay to switch things up and tweak the recipes until you find what's best for your hair. Remember, you determine what regular means in your deep conditioning regimen but it MUST be regular. You need to remain diligent and consistent during the harsher weather months as they cause hair to dry out faster and become frizzier. There are plenty of deep conditioning treatments you can buy at your local drugstore or beauty supply outlet, but sometimes a homemade conditioner will do just as good, and sometimes better. It also helps that you don't have to leave your house to get them either. Keep the staples available.

Just to recap about use of these recipes:

Always start on a freshly washed hair, preferably pre pooed as well, prior to applying a deep conditioner. Move the mixture from your tips up to the root, giving the treatment time to penetrate those exposed ends. Once it's fully applied, place a cap or bag of some sort over it. Wrap it with a towel, put on a heating cap, or sit under the dryer for 20 – 30 minutes. The heat will lift the cuticle in the follicle allowing the hair shaft to absorb the mixture. Remember not to overdo it. An hour or less for deep conditioning will prevent the hair from becoming over saturated, limp, and weak. Now for lighter treatments to help you refresh your styles until your next wash day take a look at the following Leave-In Conditioner recipes.

LEAVE IN CONDITIONERS & OTHER OUT OF THE BOX MOISTURIZERS

So your wash day has come and gone, your hairstyle is tired and can use some reviving; why not refresh with a leave-in conditioner? The following recipes and suggestions should help carry those coils until your next wash day.

1. **DAILY MOISTURIZER** – A much more simpler recipe that's used to stretch the conditioner and other leave

in conditioning products you may have left but not enough for a full use. This can be used as a great moisturizer as well as an amazing detangler using some of those staples you're supposed to be keeping in the house now.

Ingredients:

½ cup of your left over conditioner

1 spray bottle

10 – 15 drops of any essential oil (tea tree, thyme, lavender, peppermint, etc.)

2 – 3 tablespoons Extra Virgin Olive Oil (this can be cut with another oil or substituted out completely)

2 ¼ cup of water

Directions:

Get the ingredients into the spray bottle. Shake it up. Spritz and go! Revive those curls in a few minutes or less.

2. JOJOBA AND MINT CONDITIONER – Another go to conditioner that is easy peasy when it comes to homemade products. All you need are the following:

Ingredients:

1 Spray Bottle (any new spray bottle will do, but if using an old one, make sure it was used for hair care products or ingredients you would use in your hair care recipes. Don't use bottles that once held cleaning chemicals or anything like that.)

2 tablespoons Jojoba Oil

¼ cup Water

3 – 6 drops of Peppermint essential oil

Directions:

Pour the contents into the spray bottle. Shake well to blend and pow!

Spray onto dry, dull hair.

It smells wonderful and works wonderfully compared to similar leave-ins on the market. Please be careful when adding the peppermint oil as too much will overwhelm your senses and those around you. Dilute, dilute, dilute that peppermint oil to ensure it isn't a hindrance rather than an essential tool to help your hair remain luxuriously soft and smelling delight.

3. **Ease the Frizz Coconut Oil** – When your locks are misbehaving try a dollop or two of some coconut oil as a leave in conditioner. When you smooth it onto wet hair, you'll get an amazing sheen, softness for days, and some body to otherwise limp locks. It's too simple to mess up so give it a try.

Ingredients:

½ cup coconut oil

Directions:

Apply to wet or dry hair as necessary to get the desired feel you're looking for.

So simple and easy to use and notice ... NO blender.

4. SOOTHING ANTI DANDRUFF LEAVE IN CONDITIONER – So what happens when your itchy and flaky scalp won't let you be great? Fight back with this leave in conditioner that will soothe the irritated skin and treat your coils like the luxurious strands they are. It's a laundry list of ingredients but it is a sure fire treatment that will fight those flaky patches.

Ingredients

1 cup of warm water

1/3 cup of Aloe Vera liquid

2 Tablespoons coconut oil

2 Tablespoons lemon juice

6 vitamin E oil pills

15 – 20 drops of thyme oil

10 – 15 drops of tea tree oil (If you're getting close to the 10 drops and the smell is overwhelming; STOP. The smell of this oil is very, very potent and while you may not mind, the burning eyes and nostrils of others around you just might. So use this oil with caution. While it has great antiseptic and healing properties, restraint is more essential than the oil itself.)

½ cup of coconut milk

1 spray bottle (Again, these can be bought new for very cheap, or use an old spray bottle that once contained hair care products)

Directions:

Now get all those wonderful liquids into that spray bottle, close and shake shake shake. Shake your groove thang. Seriously, shake the bottle before every use, spray into your hair, and go on about your day while this concoction treats your itchy scalp; saving you from those little white flakes that drop and rest on your shoulders and everywhere else your hair shakes free.

5. **SHEA BUTTER CREAM** – This delightful emollient can be used to stretch your regular conditioners into an even better leave in treatment. The shea

butter conditioning cream can be used as a standalone ingredient with a little bit of water to stretch it or add it an existing conditioner to really prolong its usage. The shea butter conditioning cream can usually be found in any beauty supply store or the ethnic hair care section at your local drug store. It's usually a peachy pink color, super soft, and priced around five dollars.

Ingredients:

1 cup Shea Butter Cream Conditioner

¼ cup your leftover conditioner

Enough water to fill

1 spray bottle

Directions:

Mix in the bottle and shake it like a Polaroid picture. This moisturizing leave in will leave your hair soft and lush as you make your way through your day. It lasts longer than the store bought conditioner and it saves some money.

6. CLARIFYING CONDITIONER – Another simple concoction to help your hair hold on to your love and condition between wash days. It only contains one ingredient and that is good ole apple cider vinegar. ACV has long been touted as the end all, be all, to household and health uses. It can clean your toilet and your digestive track. It can help you lose weight while also cleansing and conditioning your hair.

Ingredients:

½ cup apple cider vinegar

½ cup water

Directions:

Keep it simple, and mix equal parts vinegar to water. This should be applied before conditioning and after shampoo, so that once you rinse your conditioner, you rinse away the odor of the vinegar. As wonderfully amazing this may be for your strands, smelling like vinegar may not be the most pleasant way to spend your day.

5. Leave In Detangler – As mentioned earlier, take care to the items listed in these recipes as you may be allergic to something. If you are allergic, omit that item, and if you find out you're allergic to something, seek medical attention immediately. You can also try an alternative like vegetable glycerin. It's an all - natural product that you can find in most drug stores and you may want to keep it on hand with the rest of those staple ingredients.

Ingredients:

1/2 cup vegetable glycerin

2 cups of water

1 spray bottle

Make sure to dilute the glycerin with 4 times as much water as glycerin.

Directions:

Mix and spray onto hair. The mixture is easy to make and often soothing to delicate skin. If you're prone to breakouts and are just sensitive to products, this may be the mixture for you to try.

7. ANTI - FRIZZ HOMEMADE LEAVE IN CONDITIONER – Another anti – frizz treatment that's great for your hair and easy on the wallet. Get your curls to

shine in all of their glory with this
moisture locking conditioner.

Ingredients:

3 tablespoons Jojoba Oil

3 tablespoons Sweet Almond Oil

1 teaspoon Vegetable Glycerin

10 – 15 drops of Rosemary Oil

2 – 3 cups warm water

1 spray bottle (alter the amount of water to the
size of the spray bottle)

Directions:

Mix into the bottle, and shake it like a salt shaker. Spray onto your hair and be prepared for your hair to sing your praises as it lays just the way you like it, just the way it's supposed to.

OUT OF THE BOX MOISTURIZERS

8. ROOIBOS TEA RINSE – I know you're probably reading this thinking how absurd it must be to rinse your hair with tea, but you'd be wrong, and a tea rinse is great! Don't knock it until you try it but chilled tea poured onto the hair will work wonders on your curly coils. The best tea to use is Rooibos tea, which is also known as red tea. It is great for encouraging moisture, illuminating shine, and clarifying your hair of all those pesky things it picks up from the environment and product buildup between your wash days. It curbs your cravings for sweets, gives your skin an illustrious glow, and battles acne like a champion.

Ingredients:

2 Rooibos or red tea tea bags

2 cups water

Directions:

You can brew the tea bags in the 2 cups of water and allow it to cool before applying it. Or let the bags steep (just leave it sitting in the water) for 45 minutes. The tea MUST be COOL before you apply it to your hair. Please, please, please do not use scalding hot tea on your scalp or any part of your body for that matter. Don't even drink it that hot.

Once cool, apply the tea rinse to your hair. Pour it slowly over your hair so you can maneuver the fast moving liquid around to coat your hair thoroughly. Rinse with warm water and then condition afterward.

7. **BUTTER** – A lustrous emollient but what about the regular butter, churned from cream, that sits in your refrigerator? Yes, actual butter, and even its margarine alternatives can work as a moisturizing conditioner in a pinch. You may want to pop some popcorn, or butter some biscuits while this fatty goodness sits in your hair, for 30 minutes to an hour, but your tresses will glisten and retain moisture like a cactus in a desert. Give this recipe a try if you don't want to use the butter on its own:

Ingredients:

½ cup or 4 tablespoons butter (This really can be any butter, from Country Crock, to shea butter, to mango butter. Any butter you love will do because it just so happens the butter you cook with can be used if you run out of the others.)

2 tablespoons mayonnaise

3 tablespoons honey

3 tablespoons almond oil

Directions:

Blend the ingredients together in a bowl. You may want to warm the butters to make them more susceptible to hand mixing. Once they're combined, lather the elixir onto your hair and scalp. Cover for 20 minutes and rinse with warm to cool water.

Dry and style as usual.

8. VITAMIN E CAPSULES - Have you ever taken a walk down the vitamin aisle and notice those clear, yellow hued, vitamin E capsules? Have you ever thought to use them in your hair? Maybe, the next time you pass them in the store, you should pick up a bottle. Once you get the pills home, open about 10 – 20 of these pills into a bowl or glass jar. Scoop out the paste and spread onto your hair and scalp. The plain oil should be available as well in case you don't wanna rip open a bunch of pills. You are going to let this paste sit in your hair for about 2 to 3 hours. You can use this as an overnight treatment and it's super simple to do, especially if you have the time to do it. If you do choose to do this as an overnight treatment, be sure to wear a cap under your scarf or bonnet in order to save your pillowcases and sheets from any greasy run off. Oil stains are a pain to remove. Make sure to rinse your hair well in the morning to get the paste out and style as normal. Here's an easy recipe to juice this up a bit:

Ingredients:

20 Vitamin E Capsules or ¼ cup Vitamin E oil

2 tablespoons castor or Jamaican black castor oil

2 tablespoons coconut oil

1/3 cup cocoa butter

Directions:

Mix the oils and butter into a paste and apply to your hair from tip to root. Let the mixture sit in your hair for half hour or overnight. Make sure to cover to let the oils penetrate your strands.

Rinse extremely well with warm to hot water. Blot dry your hair and style as usual.

WRAPPING IT UP

Caring for your natural hair should not break the bank, and cheap solutions should not dilute the quality of your hair care regimen. These recipes are merely suggestions to stretch your products, stretch your budget, but most importantly stretch your hair to its full potential. Use what you like, substitute what you don't, and find what your hair likes the best. No two head are the same, but the next few suggestions will help along with the upkeep of your new hair care routine, especially if you have colder and harsh fall and winter seasons. Keeping your hair moisturized is critical to managing your hair and minimizing damage. Some simple night time tactics will help keep your hair soft and conditioned, even when you don't want or shouldn't go out with moist hair.

Satin or Silk At Night Feels Just Right

Silk on silk on silk on silk. No it's not a trendy rap song but something to take into consideration when wrapping your hair up at night. Perform your nightly hair treatment using some of the staples listed above. A liquid, oil, and conditioner / emollient method will suffice, or the LOC method as it is otherwise known as. Once you are LOC'ed, wrap your hair with a silk/ satin scarf, slip on a satin bonnet, and sleep on silk or satin pillowcases. This will keep your hair extra juicy and protected as you sleep through the night.

It's All About Love, Peace, & Hair Grease

For the rare occurrence when that cream, butter, or other emollient doesn't want to absorb or work with your coils, go back to hair grease. A little goes a long way, but using those Softee greases, with coconut oil, Indian hemp, and/or other essential nutrients and oils can take the place of your sealant when you're in a bind. You can layer the grease on top of the cream rather than a full substitution as that may require an impromptu wash day or night.

Hot & Humid Ain't Just for Summer Time

If your bedroom is all nice and toasty, and your snug as a bug in a rug; that heat may be drying out the air while dream away peacefully. Turn on a humidifier that will replenish the much needed moisture being sapped from the air by the heat.

Seal the Deal on Wet Hair

The hair doesn't have to be dripping wet, but it should be damp when you touch it. Wet it real good, a cup to cup and a half of water should do the trick. Blot your hair with a T - shirt or microfiber towel to absorb the excess. This is a technique to revitalize those dry, third day, twist or braid outs. Follow up with an oil of your choice, coconut or Jamaican black castor oil should do nicely, and then twist or braid your hair up to trap that moisture inside overnight. Remember to double and triple up on that satin or silk after performing this quick treatment.

WHY MOISTURE HELPS RETAIN LENGTH

There is a perceived notion, on natural sites and blogs, that reducing dry hair is the track to full, long, luxuriously healthy hair. This is a half -truth, and while there are certain times where moisture helps in the manageability of natural hair, there some times where moisture has no role. So here's a quick summary of why retaining moisture should not be your solitary goal when caring for your kinky coils.

One of the biggest misconceptions out there is that moisture helps your hair grow. It does not. Your hair will not grow due to solely moisturizing. Hair growth is not influenced at all by the level of water being held in your hair shafts. Your diet, genetics, and hair growth cycle influence growth. Even if you don't have the best eating habits, your hair will still grow at a normal rate but if it's depleted or starving of protein, your hair will either fall out, slow down, or just stop growing. Helping your hair grow faster doesn't require it to be moisturized, but moisturized hair does help retain growth.

Retaining the growth of your strands can definitely be assisted by keeping them moist.

Moisture in the strand is really there to alleviate the damage hair may sustain while washing, styling, and just everyday wear and tear. The less damage your strands sustain mean the longevity is increased substantially as these strands won't have to be trimmed or cut.

Styling your hair, from standard combing and brushing (although many prefer to use their fingers to lessen the stress on your follicles), to styling your own hair freely or in some kind of protective style. Braiding or twisting the hair while dry will encourage that snap, crackle, and pop that will make you cringe as the broken shafts fall to the floor around you. You're going to shed hair, that's inevitable and apart of the process, but there's no need to amplify it. A quick spritz or light dousing with a bit of water can go a long way when styling as it allows the hair to be manipulated a lot easier without as much breakage.

However, no matter how soft you get your hair or how lovely it looks after a lustrous moisturizing treatment, you cannot eliminate dry hair. Accept it. The sooner you accept this, the less chance you have in being disappointed when your hair starts to revert after your regular conditioning treatments stop or become fairly irregular. Naturally dry hair will always be dry hair because these treatments and recipes you implement are only temporary. For a few naturalistas, using certain products like a drying shampoo can result in abnormally dry hair but removing that product should allow moisture to be restored. Yet, the vast majority of people with kinky, curly, coiled hair will tend to have dry tresses. The main reason for the emphasis on having a "regular" (remember you determine what's regular for you) hair care conditioning routine is because keeping the hair moisturized with water and oils, constantly penetrating the shaft, is a job that has to be repeated regularly, often times weekly, because hair reverts back to its default parched state from the moisturized state you've been implementing. Don't feel like keeping up with the constant bombardment of water onto your locks? Let the environment do it, by going somewhere nice and humid so your hair can absorb the water in the air all on its own. Some foreign beach sounds nice right about now.

Also keep in mind that moisture has a direct correlation to shrinkage. Even when you think your hair is short and stubby and being super stubborn, it may be suffering from shrinkage. Afrocentric hair has a tendency to shrink up to

70% from its actual length. Moisture encourages your hair to remain in its natural, tightly, coiled, curl pattern which will work against you if you are trying to show off its amazing length and progress. Take it easy on the water when you want to adorn your hair with particular styles like a blow out, or twists. It's been found that using less water, and other moisturizers, while wearing these styles prolong the wear ability.

Again, regular is what you deem to be regular so moisture routines are going to vary. Maintenance for moisturized hair has no set formula or schedule. Some people may find they only need to wash, condition, and apply a leave in weekly. For some other curl girls, misting the hair while applying a butter, oil, or other emollient once or twice a day may do it. There is also alternating products and practices, like shampooing one wash day a month and then for every other wash day only using conditioner. Finding the best routine that works for you, your time and your hair is the best bet to strengthening and retaining moisture.

Overall, the recipes and information found in this book are here as a guide, not a strict how-to manual. Trial and error is the best way to find out what works best for you and your curly coils. Don't be afraid to try new things and alter these recipes based off of what you learn about yourself going through your hair care process.

Remember to blend fruits in a blender to eliminate chunks that will stick to your hair and annoy you to the highest levels of irritability. Substitute components out that you don't like, or are allergic to, to make the recipe work for you. Let your conditioner do the job you made it for. Let it sit for an average of 30 minutes before rinsing, unless it's a henna treatment. Do NOT deep condition overnight as too much moisture will do more harm to your hair than good. Super saturating your hair will leave you in a wet mess, while your hair appears to be limp, heavy, and weak. Apply heat to your butters prior to mixing so they are workable. Apply heat to your deep conditioners to amplify the process and encourage moisture retention. Do NOT rinse conditioners containing eggs with hot water and do not mix eggs with any hot ingredients, as you're liable to end up with a delectable scrambled egg entrée on your head. Heating up these recipes prior to using them is recommended but do not use or handle these products if they're piping hot. Burning your scalp, or any other body part, isn't worth the perfection of a perfectly juicy twist out.

Keep the staples in the house so if you run out of your store bought conditioner, or you just want to try something out, you can whip something up in a pinch. The staples are listed above, but a few are, water, aloe vera juice, extra virgin olive oil, coconut oil, shea butter, mayonnaise, and/ or cocoa butter. Having a few of these ingredients lying around can mix up an amazing pre-poo, deep conditioner, or leave in conditioner.

The most important thing to remember as you find what works best for you, is that you are unique. Comparing your journey to another person's will set you up for failure every single time. Take cues, tips, and techniques from others but remain vigilant in maintaining your hair, your way. Don't judge your own growth cycle or hair appearance because it is naturally beautiful. Give yourself time to learn you, and what your coily strands love, as nothing happens overnight. Love your hair and the scalp it grows out of. If you're going to compare anything, compare your hair today to where it was 6 months ago, or a year ago, or even a week ago. Track your progress. Pay attention to your triumphs and even more attention to the fails. It is a never ending journey to achieve a healthy head of hair and the most important part of that journey is a healthier you.

Conclusion

Thank you again for reading *Natural Hair Recipes For Moisture and Growth*. And congratulations on taking a step in the direction of healthier hair.

The next step is to buy get started making some recipes.

Thank You!

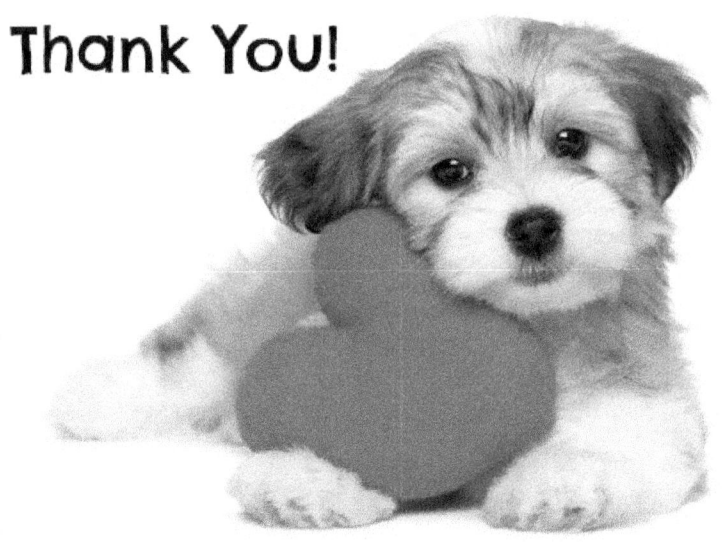

Finally, if you enjoyed this book, then I'd like to ask you for a favor, would you be kind enough to leave a review for this book? It'd be greatly appreciated!

Your review will give me feedback on the book, tips on how to improve it or a pat on the back for a job well done. Plus, it helps others find the book.

Thank you and good luck!

Preview of 'Natural Hair Growth Secrets'

Chapter 1: How To Care For Natural Hair

The best way to grow your hair is to take very good care of it. If you procrastinate and don't take the proper care, your hair will not grow any longer.

We all get lazy at times. Sometimes when it's time to do my twists over, I simply don't feel like it. But when it comes down to it, **you will get out of it what you put into it.**

If you use the methods in this book, your hair will grow, and it will grow consistently long. It's up to you to apply what you learn.

Treatments

To grow your hair you will need to treat it. How often will vary depending on your hair style. But ultimately you should be treating your hair every 2 weeks.

When I say treatments I mean pre-pooing, shampooing, washing, conditioning, hot oil treatments, and trimming.

Pre-Poo

A pre-poo is what you do before shampooing your hair. This prepares your hair for the shampooing which can be very harsh and strip your hair.

A pre-poo is optional, but I recommend you do it because it makes your hair much easier to untangle.

<u>What you will need:</u> a moisturizing conditioner, natural oils such as extra virgin olive oil or coconut oil, shower cap or plastic shopping bag

A pre-poo is pretty similar to a deep condition, but less complicated. The purpose of the pre-poo is to prepare your hair to be washed.

Step 1: Separate your hair into manageable sections (4-8 depending on length). Do this by sectioning off your hair into ponytails, knots, or twists.

Step 2: Take out one section of your hair that you want to work on first. Grab your conditioner or natural oils or a mixture of both and apply it to the section. Once the section is finished put it back into a ponytail.

Step 3: Apply the oils and conditioner generously to the section by either spraying or rubbing it onto your hair. If applying directly from the bottle into your hands-- make sure you're making a root to tip motion.

Step 4: Repeat the process with all sections of your head.

Step 5: Put on a shower cap or plastic shopping bag to enclose the conditioner and oils. Let sit for 45min-2hours.

Step 6: Take your hair out of the shower cap or plastic bag and, while it's still in its sections, rinse it out using cold water. This will seal in the moisture and close the cuticles.

Step 7: Go on to your shampoo routine.

Visit <u>www.naturalhairmaster.com/resources/</u> to continue reading Natural Hair Recipes

Check Out My Other Books

Below you'll find some of my other popular natural hair books that are popular on Amazon and Kindle as well. Simply click on the links below to check them out.

The Beginners Guide To Natural Hair: How To Begin Your Natural Hair Journey Today

Natural Hair Growth Secrets: How To Grow Natural Hair Long

Natural Hair Recipes: Do It Yourself Natural Hair Products

Natural Hair Transitioning: The Complete Guide To Transitioning From Relaxed To Natural Hair

The Big Chop: Guide To Starting Your Natural Hair Journey From Scratch

If the links do not work, for whatever reason, you can simply search for these titles on the Amazon website to find them.

Natural Hair Checklist & Journal [FREE]

Our printable checklist provides you with a list of everything you'll need to begin your natural hair journey.

Take it with you on the go, it can be downloaded on any device.

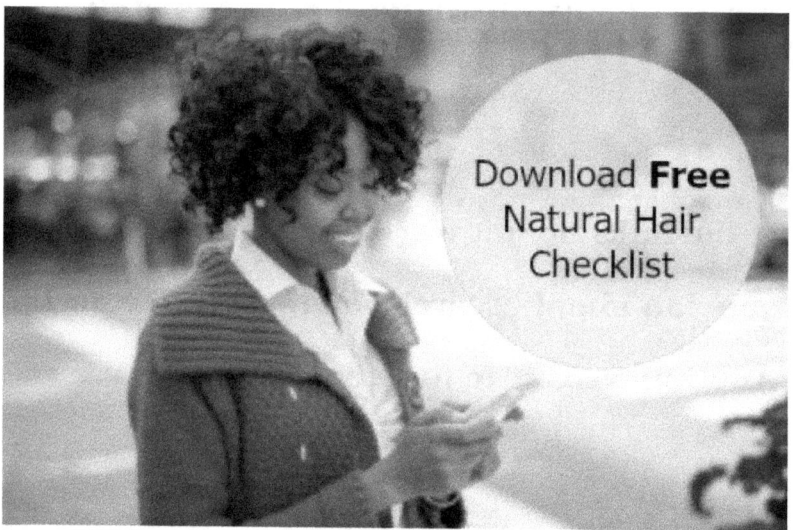

As an added **BONUS** you'll receive our **Natural Hair Journey Journal**. A digital journal where you can track your experiences of growth, recipes, and more.

www.naturalhairmaster.com/naturalhairchecklistandjournal

About The Author

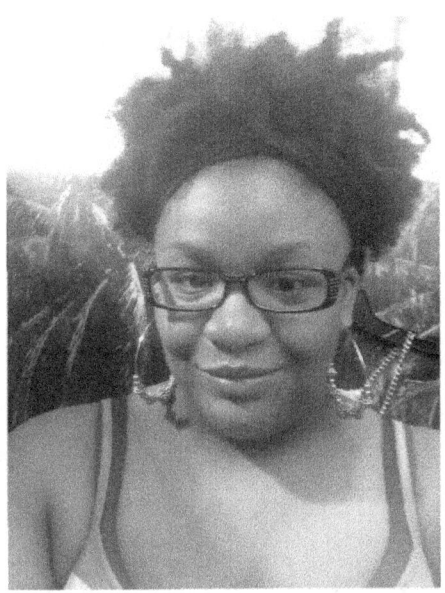

Hello my name is Argena Hall and I'm here because I am passionate about helping women on their natural hair journey.

I know what it is like to be confused about where to start and not knowing what products you need and how to style your own natural hair.

It wasn't long ago that I was searching online for natural hair tutorials and trying to figure out where to start.

Then I discovered a way to start going natural and doing my own hair.

It hasn't always been easy. I have run into problems like not knowing what twisting creams to use or if I should get the "big chop".

Now I've been natural for three whole years! And my hair has been growing like crazy.

And now I want to help you to get the same results. The first step is simple, download my free beginner's natural hair checklist to ensure you purchase the right products to get started with you natural hair journey.